Weight Loss & WELLNESS
the SV Ayurveda Way

STEP-up YOUR SUGAR & FAT
METABOLISM

BY VAIDYA R.K. MISHRA • LISSA COFFEY

Weight Loss & Wellness the SV Ayurveda Way
Step-up Your Sugar & Fat Metabolism

Copyright © 2016 Vaidya R.K. Mishra and Lissa Coffey
Published by
Adishakti LLC
11856 Balboa Blvd.
Suite 333
Granada Hills, California
91344
U S A

All rights reserved. No part of this book may be reproduced in whole or in part without written permission from the publisher, except by reviewers who may quote brief excerpts in connection with a review in a newspaper, magazine, or electronic publication; no parts of this book be reproduced, stored in a retrieval system, or transmitted in any form or by any means electronic, mechanical, photocopying, recording, or other, without written permission from the publisher.

ISBN: 978-1-61021-001-0

For the Divine Mother

Table of Content

Introduction	5
Chapter 1: Ayurveda: What You Need to Know	9
Chapter 2: Metabolize Your Fat!	24
Chapter 3: Metabolize Your Sugar!	51
Chapter 4: The Art of Eating for Optimal Digestion	73
Chapter 5: The Importance of Protein	76
Chapter 6: Recipes	95
Scientific References	113
About the Authors	117
Aknowledgements	120
Resources	121

Introduction

If you go on Amazon and do a search using the word "metabolism" you'll get more than 50,000 results in a number of different categories. There is so much out there telling us we need to lose weight, burn fat, boost metabolism, cleanse toxins, balance hormones, diet, jumpstart, rev-up or slim down! The amount of content is mind-boggling. Yet the lack of accurate information is a big problem when we're really trying to help ourselves, and not cause more harm to an already over-burdened digestive system.

Metabolism is the process the body goes through to convert food into energy. The body needs this energy for everything it does, whether strenuous or restful. A person's metabolism is determined by many factors, including genetics, gender, age, hormones, body type, and activity level. Men typically have a higher metabolism rate than women. Ideally we want the body to have a metabolism that provides for us all the energy we need to do all the activities and work we want to do.

When the body's metabolism is too slow, or not functioning as efficiently as it should, we may experience symptoms such as low blood pressure, a slow pulse, fatigue or apathy, constipation, dry skin, weakness, excess body fat (particularly belly fat), headaches, and an increased sensitivity to cold. There are many reasons that our metabolism might be out of whack – including eating unhealthy foods, or fasting, or lack of exercise.

Diabetes is a chronic disease where the body does not produce, or doesn't properly regulate insulin. Insulin is a hormone that helps the body to store and use energy that we get from sugar, starches and other foods. Without enough insulin, unmetabolized sugar, or glucose, builds up in the blood causing damage to the body and its systems. Unmetabolized sugar gets stored as fat.

According to the Centers for Disease Control and Prevention (CDC), 29 million people in the United States have diabetes. That's almost 10%! A study published by JAMA (Journal of the American Medical Association) says that nearly 50% of all adults living in the United States either have diabetes or pre-diabetes, a condition where a person has elevated blood sugar and is at risk for developing diabetes. The CDC says that the leading cause of diabetes is obesity, and that in the past 30 years both the rates of obesity and diabetes have been rising.

Stress is also an issue. Stress leads the body to increase production of the hormone cortisol. Cortisol gets into the bloodstream and inhibits insulin.

Menopause is another factor that can slow the metabolism. As estrogen levels decrease, the body tries to compensate by storing fat around the belly. Slow metabolism and weight gain feed off of each other and we get caught in a downward spiral.

So then we don't feel good. And when we don't feel good, we get depressed, and we don't feel like we look good. We wonder if we'll ever feel fit or fabulous again. Clearly, something is wrong.

What's wrong is that we are eating the wrong foods, cooking them the wrong way, eating them the wrong way, and therefore not metabolizing our foods properly. We're working too much, and too hard, and not taking care to balance our lives with the rest and peace that both the body and mind crave. This causes a terrible strain on the entire system that shows up as dis-ease, or disease. As much as we can blame food companies for putting unhealthy food at our disposal, it really is our own responsibility to choose what, when, and how we eat. Isn't it time for us to get into better habits? To have an awareness of the harm that we are doing to ourselves?

Fortunately, Ayurveda has an answer for us. In this centuries old science lies the ancient wisdom that we need right now to get our bodies back into balance and functioning as optimally as they are meant to. This book is meant to provide you will all the information you need to help your body metabolize both fat and sugar the way it is meant to. Now you have the information in your hands. And now you know that your health is in your hands. It is up to you to take the necessary steps to change your habits so that you can be the healthiest and happiest YOU possible! You'll feel fit and fabulous – and you'll look fit and fabulous, too!

CHAPTER 1
Ayurveda: What You Need to Know

If you are familiar with yoga or meditation, you have probably heard of Ayurveda. The word "Ayurveda" comes from Sanskrit. It is broken down into two parts: "Ayu" meaning "life" and "Veda" meaning science, or unchanging knowledge. Ayurveda is literally "The Science of Life" and its roots go back more than 5,000 years to ancient India. The official "textbook" of Ayurveda is the Charak Samhita. These writings contain everything we need to know to establish and maintain the perfect health that we are meant to have.

"Life" has so many definitions, even within Ayurveda. In SVAyuveda we follow one specific definition of Ayu, and that is *Deha Prana Samyoge Ayu.* This translates to: "Life is Prana: pranic energy, and cosmic energy vibrating through our nadis, or channels." The Prana circulating in the body is what makes us alive. When Prana stops circulating, the Jivatman, or the soul, leaves the body and we die.

Cosmic energy is energy that comes from our environment through many channels, the primary being the organs of our senses: our eyes, ears, nose, skin, and mouth. This is how we experience the external world. This is also how we take in the food and water that goes to nourish the body. So food and water are important sources of pranic, or life-giving, energy. SV Ayurveda says that our food should be full of Prana, and our water should not be lacking in Prana.

Food is an overall sensory experience. We see it, so it should look appetizing, colorful, and beautiful. We hear it when we snap the fresh vegetables, and when the food sizzles as it's cooking. We smell the wonderful aroma coming from fresh food, and even more when we cook it. You know how a good meal fills up the house with wonderful smells! We feel the texture of food with our mouths and our teeth – the texture should be pleasant and appealing. And of course, we taste the food, and it should be delicious!

Feed Prana to your body in these ways:

- By breathing. When we get scared we tend to hold our breath, which really only makes things worse.

We need oxygen to think! Sometimes we get so rattled that we forget to breathe, and when we finally take that breath we get clarity. When we're angry and people tell us to calm down and take a breath, that's really good advice. The Prana that we take in through the breath helps the mind and body to operate efficiently.

- By being in a good, natural environment. The quality of air that we breathe impacts the body. Too often we're in crowded cities full of pollution, in airplanes with stale, dry air, or indoors where we have air-conditioned or heated air. We function best out in nature where the air is pure and clean. The colors of nature, blue sky, green trees, bright flowers, are healing for our eyes. The sunlight feels good on our skin and helps to match our internal time clock to the circadian rhythm of nature. The primordial sounds of nature, birds, wind, water, are soothing to our ears. All of this helps to bring Prana to the body.

- By eating homemade organic food. Remember how Grandmother's homemade soup used to make you feel so good? That's because it was made with love. When we make food at home we know exactly which ingredients go into the recipe, and into the body. Cooking and eating in a settled, calm environments helps food to be digested most efficiently as well.

- By drinking fresh spring water. 55-60% of the body is made up of water, so doesn't it make sense to replace water that leaves our body with pure water? And yet, so many people consume soda, sugary, or artificially sweetened drinks as their main source of liquid. Research has shown a link between soda and both weight gain, and diabetes, so clearly, drinking soda is a bad idea. We not only need pure water in our diet, we need the Prana that comes from water for the body to function optimally.

The body needs pranic support from all of these sources.

There are three components to Prana:

- **Soma** comes to us with lunar energy - it is the raw material in food.

- **Agni** comes to us from solar energy – this is the power of transforming the raw material into the essences of what the body needs.

- **Marut** comes to us from the energy of space and air. It is the etheric energy that maintains the intelligence of the body while circulating the Agni, or fire energy, to where it needs to go within the body. Marut knows which organ or system needs which nutrient and when.

Pranic energy circulates throughout the body every moment, 24/7. It must for us to be alive. The combination of the body plus circulating Prana is life.

The Three Pillars of Life

According to Ayurveda, there are three pillars of a healthy life. The Charak Samhita says *Trayahupasstambha Ahar Nidra Brahamcharyashcha (Three subpillars of life: food, sleep, following the laws of nature).* The first pillar is Food, Ahar. This means that we must eat food full of Prana, "intelligent" food.

The second pillar of health is Sleep, Nidra. This means proper sleep, not just the quantity of sleep you get, but also the quality of sleep you get. And it is also about having a balance between rest and activity. We need this balance in life – it can't just be work, work, and more work all the time. We need to balance work with periods of rest and play.

The third pillar of health, brahamcharya, is often mistranslated as celibacy, and that is not the correct meaning of the word. The true meaning is "following the laws of nature." The sun is brightest at midday, and our digestion is strongest then, so that is the time when we should eat our largest meal of the day. When the sun rises, this signals that nature is waking up, so we need to wake up then as well. It is important to get to bed before 10:00 pm. There is an entire Ayurvedic daily routine, or Dinyacharya, that we can follow for maximum health benefits. (see Chapter 2).

You can see that food is essential to our health. This is the very first tenet in SV Ayurveda. The Sakavanshi Ayurveda lineage has its history documented in the Puranas, and Vaidya Mishra is from that lineage. It has a little bit of a different approach than mainstream Ayurveda in that it focuses on food so much that followers might feel overwhelmed with all the knowledge. But the people who follow the SV Ayurveda plan always say that they feel very fortunate to have found it.

The Three Types of Food

Food should be wholesome and natural, organic and fresh. This is why it is important that you make your food at home, so that you can control the ingredients, and you know exactly what is in each dish. Most every restaurant out there makes food is acidic. They use bad oils, bad salt, synthetic vinegar, leftovers, and frozen foods. And they often use microwave ovens. Raw frozen foods are fine, but once a food is cooked it should not be frozen. Freezing foods causes the enzymes to change. You can see that the color of the food changes – that is because of oxidation. When oxidation happens free radicals, or toxins are present – and that can bring on much stress and disease to the body, including cancer.

For the same reason we don't want to eat leftovers. There are some foods we can keep in the refrigerator – milk or yogurt for example. But any processed foods kept in the refrigerator will begin to oxidize, and that's not good. It doesn't seem possible with all of our modern day technology, but that's the reality. The *Bhagavad Gita, chapter 17* has a passage that explains this. Lord Krishna says to Arjuna "even the good food (the Sattvic food) after four hours becomes Rajasic. After that is becomes Tamasic (bad food)." Rajasic food is food that has lost its freshness, its energy. If we describe Sattvic food as intelligent food, then Rajasic food is dumb food. There's still some Prana there, but not nearly as much as in the fresh food. And then Tamasic food has no Prana – it's basically just a mass lump of stuff – it's dead food. This isn't something we want to put into the body if we have any choice at all.

Choose food that is freshly made. If you make something for lunch, then want to eat it again for dinner, that's fine. But don't leave it overnight. The longer you leave the food the less Prana it has in it. The freezer kills Prana in cooked foods and the microwave kills Prana as well. No Prana means no nourishment.

Intelligent Foods, Intelligent Cooking

Sattvic food is vibrant; it feeds the cellular system, the mind, and the light of the soul. Sattvic food tastes delicious, and is satisfying to you the mind and body while also giving a sense of bliss. So how do we know which foods to choose, which foods are the most sattvic?

After you eat sattvic food you feel comfortable and happy. If you feel tired or less happy after you eat then the food was not sattvic. This is an important reason why we need to cook at home, where we can control the ingredients and we know exactly what is going into our meals. You'll find some wonderful recipes in this book, and Vaidya Mishra has more recipes up on his website and YouTube channel.

 http://www.YouTube.com/SVAHealth

The SV Ayurveda lineage focuses on the channels of the body. This is something that modern nutritional science doesn't talk about. In the body there are large physical channels, such as the esophagus or the intestine. There are also smaller physical channels, some so tiny that they can only be seen with a microscope. SV Ayurveda says that we should not eat any food that clogs these channels. Why? These physical channels help to transform the nutrients in food and direct them to the appropriate places where they are needed in the body. The channels also separate out any toxins that are present, and eliminate them. When we eat food that clogs the channels we interfere with the channels' ability to transform the food, nourish the body, and eliminate the toxins.

Channel clogging foods include larger beans, such as kidney, lima and pinto beans. Also soybeans, so this includes tofu. These beans have larger, tougher molecules. If you are working hard physically on a regular basis, you can digest the larger beans more easily. If you're not very physically active, choose to eat small beans or some of the many varieties of lentils: yellow mung, green mung, or red lentils. Lentils and beans are both in the legume family. Lentils are high in protein and fiber and low in fat. They are also high in iron, phosphorus and potassium.

Winter squashes, including butternut squash, acorn squash, and pumpkin fall into the category of channel-clogging. Avoid eating winter squash. Instead, choose from among the many varieties of Summer Squash, including zucchini, yellow squash, and Pattypan Squash.

The larger sized bananas also clog the channels. The smaller bananas aren't a problem, so be selective with your produce.

Nightshade plants, particularly tomato, potato, eggplant, and large peppers like red, green and yellow bell peppers, are also known to clog the channels. These vegetables are inflammatory by nature, that's how they are chemically made-up. They clog the circulatory channels, muting the digestive fire, and making it easier for the body to catch a cold, especially in the winter months.

Ayurveda advises us to digest a meal completely before eating the next meal. Even if the food we eat is sattvic, or good food, when we put more food on top of an undigested meal, this is called *Vishamagni.* Vishamagni creates semi-digestive material that is called *Ama.* Ama gets chemically charged, becomes acidic, and then turns into free radicals or elementary toxins. This creates inflammation in the organs and the overall digestive system. So Ayurveda recommends that we eat what we can digest easily. Lentils are very good for digestion and can be eaten on a daily basis.

SV Ayurveda also says that we need to avoid both onion and garlic. Many nutritionists endorse the benefits of onion and garlic and recommend people add both to their diets generously. But SVA has a very good reason why this is *not* a good idea. Garlic and onion are really meant to be medicines, not food. They contain sulfur, an antibiotic. An antibiotic is great when you are sick and you want to kill off bacteria. The problem is that when you aren't sick, you really don't want to kill off all the friendly bacteria, the probiotics that are naturally in your system for a reason. And that's exactly what happens when you eat garlic and onion. You wouldn't want to take an antibiotic every day, certainly not when you don't need one. And you shouldn't eat garlic and onion every day, either. A little bit for flavoring now and then is fine, but use it sparingly.

Modern research shows that the friendly bacteria we have in the gut is responsible for making all the essential neurotransmitters in the brain – as well as the brain chemicals that allow us to feel happy and balanced, such as dopamine, serotonin, and endorphin.

Ayurveda categorizes both garlic and onion as Tamasic. Too much garlic and onion can cause our brains to become destructive, or angry.

To help encourage the good bacteria that we need in the body and brain, SV Ayurveda recommends that we have a little bit of yogurt every day. One easy way is to make a beverage with 20% yogurt and 80% water, then add some toasted cumin, or some Mom's Masala. Mom's Masala is a signature blend of herbs that go so well with any dish, and the combination is balancing for all three doshas.

http://www.chandika.com/sva-moms-masala/

Salt is essential for the body. But there is a big difference in the quality of salt out there. Even the pink Himalayan salt that is considered to be so "gourmet" lately has a lot of sulfur in it, as well as traces of heavy metals. If you look at those pink salt crystals, you'll see that there are places in the rock with white crystals. Those white crystals are the best parts of the salt, and that's what is used to make Soma Salt. We separate out just the white part of the salt, and then powder it. This is a very cooling salt, more calcium salt than sodium and potassium. Soma Salt is delicious, and also good for you.

http://www.chandika.com/products/SVA-Soma-Salt.html

It might seem counterintuitive to include fat in your diet even though you might want to lose weight, or fat. But the body needs good fats for good health. We need good fat for the brain, and also to lubricate the channels. There are a few fats that SV Ayurveda recommends. Olive oil is one of those. The best way to use olive oil is by sprinkling it over foods, in a salad dressing for example. For cooking, particularly stir-fry, sesame oil is good. Make sure to choose filtered, or "cured" sesame oil.

The very best fat is ghee, also called clarified butter. But again, know that not all ghee is the same. Real ghee, the kind that SV Ayurveda recommends, is made from yogurt, rather than from milk. It's a long process, but it makes a big difference in the quality of the ghee. Ghee made from yogurt has all those good probiotics in it. SV Ayurveda makes "Mom's Ghee" and also several herbalized ghees all the authentic Ayurvedic way, from yogurt.

http://www.chandika.com/moms-ghee/

The Six Tastes

According to Ayurveda, there are six tastes, and it is best to have all six tastes present in each meal. The six tastes in Ayurveda are: sweet, sour, salty, bitter, pungent, and astringent. When all six tastes are present then our hunger will be satisfied and we are much more likely to stay in balance. Each taste plays a significant role in supporting the needs of our physiology.

SWEET (Madhur) Foods with a sweet taste help to build tissues and also calm the nervous system. These include natural sugars, milk, ghee, most grains (rice, wheat), and soft, juicy fruits like peaches and papaya.

SOUR (Amla) Foods with a sour taste help to increase the absorption of minerals and also to cleanse the tissues. Yogurt, cheese and fermented foods (vinegar, soy sauce, pickles) fall in this category, as well as sour fruits (lemon, lime, grapefruit).

SALTY (Lavan) Salt brings out the flavor in foods. It stimulates digestion and lubricates the tissues. The salty flavor is found in natural salt from the earth or sea.

BITTER (Tikt) The taste of bitter foods detoxifies the tissues. Bitter tastes are found in dark green leafy vegetables like spinach and kale, and various herbs and spices such as turmeric and fenugreek.

PUNGENT (Katu) The pungent taste stimulates digestion and boosts metabolism. Peppery spices like cayenne and black pepper as well as ginger and cinnamon fall into the pungent category. Chili peppers are pungent vegetables.

ASTRINGENT (Kashai) The astringent taste helps to absorb water, so it dries fat. It also helps to tighten the tissues. We find astringent taste in foods like beans and legumes, and fruits such as cranberries, pears, and pomegranates. Vegetables with the astringent taste include broccoli, artichoke, and asparagus. Quinoa also has an astringent taste.

CHAPTER 2

Metabolize Your Fat!

It seems like every time we turn on the TV or log onto the internet there is some new tablet or miracle cure that promises to get us "bikini ready" or super-model skinny. With celebrity endorsements and amazing "before and after" photos, it's easy to get pulled into whatever is being billed as the latest and greatest new "secret!" Some of these products really do get results short term, but what we don't see is that a few months later, the weight comes right back. Desperate to lose weight, we want to believe that there is something that can help. So we just hand over our money and buy the book, the bottle of tablets, the "program" or the membership. And then we get disappointed when yet again it didn't work. We end up right back where we started.

Ayurveda is different. First of all, this wealth of wisdom dates back more than 5,000 years. It's been tried and true for centuries. It deals with more than 700 herbs in detail. There are many of these herbs that can burn your fat. But Ayurveda says specifically: "Do not burn your fat." That might surprise you, but it's true! Ayurveda understands that contained within the micro-molecules of fat are materials, including calcium, which support bone tissue.

If we burn fat, how are the bones going to be nourished? We *need* good fat for so many reasons! If we really want to lose weight, we must have good fat in our diet, and not bad fat.

Besides eating homemade foods, and intelligent foods, Ayurveda has other recommendations for ways that we can support fat metabolism:

- Support the digestive system of the stomach. First of all, eat at the same time each day. Give the stomach time to digest the previous meal, and anticipate the next meal. Eat easy to digest food, and easy to digest protein. Add dark, leafy greens to your meals. Support the digestive enzymes with some spices. Ginger is a wonderful spice for digestion, and there is a lot of research to back this up. When cooking, add in some ginger, black pepper, cumin, coriander and/or turmeric. These are the best spices for digestion. If you like a little heat, add in some green chili. It's always a good idea to sprinkle some fresh lime juice on your food just before eating.

- Cut back on rice, or skip the rice altogether if you're wanting to lose weight. Ayurveda says that barley is the best grain to eat when you want to lose weight. Barley is the best grain to eat for glucose metabolism. Whole wheat is good, but opt for less wheat. Try replacing wheat with quinoa, which also has the benefits of providing protein.

- We need protein in our diet, and Ayurveda suggests paneer, an Indian cheese. This is best made at home so that it's not too heavy. Paneer is an excellent protein for vegetarians. Lentils are also very good. If you are a non-vegetarian then white meat is okay. But never eat red meat. The SV Ayurveda diet is strongly against red meat. If you have low hemoglobin and need it for a medical reason, then that is a special circumstance. But for the most part, in every day life, a vegetarian diet is recommended. If you must eat meat, just eat white meat. See Chapter 5 for more information about protein.

Seven Tissues (Dhatu) Of the Body

Ayurveda explains that the body is made up of seven kinds of tissues:

Rasa – the clear part of plasma

Rakta – blood

Mamsa – muscle

Maida – fat

Asthi – bone

Majja – bone marrow

Shukra – reproductive fluid

Each tissue feeds the next in sequence. The muscle tissue feeds the fat tissue, etc. We must eat good protein for the muscle and also for weight loss.

- Garcinia has been around for ages in Ayurveda – it is also called "Kokum" and it is used all over India. Garcinia, and particularly Garcinia flower, is one of the best ingredients for metabolizing protein and fat. You can add it to the spices when cooking as well. Vaidya Mishra has created special spice blends for each dosha that contain Garcinia making it very easy for us to get the perfect combination of spices we need for our mind/body type.

http://www.chandika.com/garcinia-masala-for-kapha/

SVA Also makes a Garcinia Tea for Weight Loss:

http://www.chandika.com/sva-garcinia-tea/

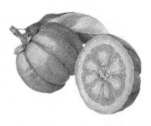

Garcinia Cambogia

- It is important to cook with spices, as spice helps make food more digestible. The whole philosophy of Ayurveda is that we must digest our food 100%, not 99%. If even just 1% of food does not get fully digested, that semi-digested material, that material, called *Ama,* and it clogs the physical channels.

When Ama stays in the body it becomes Amavisha, or toxic Ama, more commonly known as free radicals, or inflammatory chemicals. When Ama makes its way to the colon, the colon gets gassy; we feel bloated and uncomfortable. So make sure that you digest the foods you eat 100%. When food goes through the colon the colon absorbs the rest of the benefits of the food. Cumin and pomegranate are very good for enhancing absorption.

Three Parts of Digestion

The three parts of digestion we need to be mindful of are these:

- **Digestion**: Making sure that the food we eat is digested fully, 100% so that there is no Ama left behind.

- **Absorption**: Making sure the nutrients in the food have the ability to be absorbed by the various organs of the body.

- **Elimination**: Making sure that all of the waste product remaining from food leaves the body. To do this we need to get some probiotics every day so that the colon functions optimally.

Friendly bacteria play many roles that help with weight loss as well. When we eat good, fresh, foods like vegetables or grains, the friendly bacteria feed on the vitamins and minerals, giving them even more life and energy when they are infused into the body.

Have you ever noticed that when you take antibiotics you feel tired and weak? That is because the antibiotics kill the friendly bacteria, so there's nothing there to absorb the minerals and get them through the body. This is another reason to avoid onion and garlic.

The whole system must be in balance every day: Digestion, Absorption, and Elimination.

Role of the Liver

After proper absorption, the clear part of plasma, rasa, goes to the liver where it is processed. The liver is responsible for processing everything, including the rasa, the clear juice of plasma. The liver is very intelligent, even more intelligent than the brain. Why? Here is an example of the way the liver works:

Someone gets sick and needs to rehydrate the body. The doctor prescribes glucose or saline without checking the blood. However, if this person needed a blood transfusion, the doctor would always check the blood – for fear of giving the wrong type of blood to the patient.

In a family, everyone eats the same food. The liver is intelligent, and transforms that food into material that is compatible with each person's specific genomes, specific DNA, and specific blood type. As you can see, the liver is super-intelligent, and working for us all the time. So never do anything that could harm your liver. Be very careful with medications, because this puts stress on the liver. Medications are highly concentrated, processed by benzenes and hexanes that are used for extraction and as solvents. In addition, there are preservatives in medication. This is tough on the liver.

Turmeric

It is very important for the liver to be healthy so that it can work optimally for fat metabolism. The liver must break down the fat, and also clean the fat. To support the liver and all the work it has to do, the best spice is turmeric. In Ayurvedic cooking turmeric is used with everything exactly for this reason. You'll find turmeric particularly delicious in vegetable and lentil dishes.

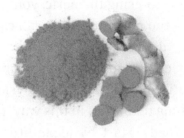

Turmeric Root and Turmeric Powder

Since turmeric is so prevalent in Indian cooking, you might wonder why Indians have so many health problems. In ancient India there weren't health problems like there are now, because everyone ate "real" turmeric. These days, most, maybe as much as 80% of the turmeric powder in Indian grocery stores, is either adulterated, or totally fake, containing no authentic turmeric. Even though you see all the nutritional facts printed on the label, the package contains tinted chalk with synthetic perfume. "Fake" turmeric will put toxins in your liver. Always make sure your turmeric is real. Vaidya Mishra sources the best turmeric from India so you can be assured that the turmeric used in the SV Ayurveda product line are up to his very high standards.

http://www.chandika.com/organic-turmeric-powder/

If you are new to using turmeric, you need to start slowly. Using too much turmeric can cause a detox crisis. In a detox crisis you may experience symptoms such as nausea, diarrhea and/or a rash on the skin. This is because the physiology is not used to flushing toxins out in this way, to the whole system overloads. Start by using little pinches of turmeric, and slowly increase the amount you add into your recipes. It is also a good idea to toast turmeric in ghee or sesame oil so that it is more easily assimilated into your system.

Turmeric comes from a root; it is a natural spice that maintains your liver's intelligence. It also helps to support cholesterol metabolism. When your cholesterol is high, a doctor will often prescribe certain medications that task your liver to create more bile, and the bile then goes into the intestine to help with cholesterol metabolism. But if you eat turmeric your cholesterol levels will naturally be good.

Besides being great for fat metabolism, turmeric is also the best armor for your immune system. Turmeric works for sugar metabolism as well, as you will discover in the pages to follow. Turmeric helps you in so many ways, and there is a lot of research to back this up.

Other Recommended Herbs for Fat Metabolism

- **Sarsaparilla** is an Indian herb that is very mild, and not heating. It is very good for fat metabolism. Use a little bit in your tea, just a few pinches. http://www.chandika.com/indian-sarsaparilla/

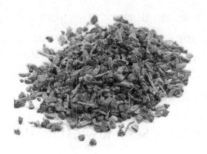

Indian Sarsaparilla

-**Fenugreek** works on both fat and glucose metabolism. Toast it in ghee a little bit to take away some of the bitter taste. After toasting you can sprinkle a little of the fenugreek powder or fenugreek seed on your food. You can also toast fenugreek with turmeric, ginger, cumin, coriander and a bit of black pepper, and then sprinkle it on food for a delicious flavor.

http://www.chandika.com/fenugreek-seeds/

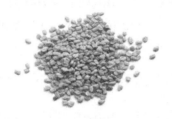

Fenugreek Seeds

Ingredients to Support Fat Metabolism

- Spices: fenugreek, turmeric, cumin, black pepper, green cardamom, curry leaf, kalaungi (black seed)

- Salt: Soma Salt

- Fats: Ghee, Sesame Oil, Olive Oil

- Lentils and Beans (Dahl): Chana, mung, Kulthi, Masoor

- Vegetables: Leafy Greens, Califlower, Broccoli, Brussels Sprouts, Lauki, Summer Squashes, Methi Leaf, Guar

- Grains: Barley, Rye

- Sweeteners: Honey, Fructose

- Dairy: Yogurt, Almond Milk

- Fruits: Apple, Cherry, Grapefruit, Pear, Prunes, Apricot

The beauty of Ayurvedic cooking is that it is healthy cooking. You enjoy the flavor and you also get the medicinal benefits from the food.

You don't have to starve yourself and deprive yourself when you want to lose fat. You have to eat good food, three meals a day and one snack. Nuts and seeds make a good snack. You can make a mixture of sunflower seeds, almonds, some dried fruits, and then soak them over night. Toss with a little bit of cumin powder, or Mom's Masala (Vaidya Mishra's signature spice blend), Soma Salt, and fresh lime juice. You can have this as a snack between lunch and dinner.

Dinyacharya

In Ayurveda, the recommended daily routine is called *Dinyacharya.* Nature has its own time-clock, and we function most optimally when we are in harmony with nature.

- Wake up at sunrise, about 6:00 A.M.

- Use the bathroom.

- Brush your teeth and tongue.

- Give yourself an Ayurvedic massage (Abhyanga – see detailed instructions below).

- Do your Yoga stretches and/or your exercise program. Also Pranayama, breathing exercises.

- Take a warm shower or bath.

- Meditate (Ideally 20-30 minutes).

- Eat a light breakfast.

- Work or study.

- Eat lunch, your largest meal of the day, at the same time each day, between noon and 1:00 P.M.

- Work or study.

- Meditate before dinner.

- Eat a light dinner, at the same time each day, preferably before 6:30 P.M.

- Take a short walk to aid digestion.

- Relax. Read. Listen to music. Visit with friends.

- Get to bed by 10:00 P.M.

If your mornings are hectic and you need to leave the house very early, you may choose to do your massage and shower in the evening. Doing so will give you an especially restful night's sleep. If you wake up hungry, as many of us do, you may choose to eat breakfast before your shower. Ayurveda will prove beneficial in whatever way it is blended into your routine. Even just adding a couple of new things into your established routine will give you a good start. There are no hard and fast rules here. Be gentle, and flexible with yourself and use this as a good guideline.

Consistency is what matters, and what will make the biggest difference. It is nice to take your time in the morning and fit in all of the Ayurvedic routine, but if you are in a hurry, it is better to do it all quickly rather than to skip it altogether. And be easy on yourself. Ayurveda is flexible, so figure out what works for you. You might not be able to do every single thing at first, but if you can do more than half, you will still see benefits. The main thing is not to stress about it. Start where you are comfortable, and grow from there.

It is important to move every single day – exercise, do yoga, walk. There is no substitute for being physically mobile. We need a minimum of 20 minutes a day of brisk walking or exercise. With today's sedentary lifestyle, where we spend most of the time either at our computer or in the car commuting to work, we need to balance with exercise to maintain the mobility in the body.

You'll also notice that Dinyacharya includes a meditation practice twice daily. You can meditate, chant, pray, spend time in silence in nature, or whatever works for you. We all need some kind of a spiritual practice for the health of our spirit.

HOME DETOX

Panchakarma (PK) in Sanskrit means "five actions." This is an age-old Ayurvedic process that dislodges and discharges accumulated toxins from the seven tissues and removes the aggravated doshas from the physiology. Many Ayurvedic clinics and spas offer this service. However, if you are eating properly, and following the daily routine, it is likely unnecessary for you to go through this whole program, which can also be costly.

However, if you are feeling sluggish, and out of balance, you may choose to do a "home detox" on your own twice a year, or three times a year maximum, at the change of the Ayurvedic seasons.

Vata Season: Fall (November through February in the Northern Hemisphere)

Kapha Season: Spring (March through June in the Northern Hemisphere)

Pitta Season: Summer (July through October in the Northern Hemisphere)

Vaidya Mishra has tailored a highly effective and easy-to-follow Home Detox Plan for you to get all the benefits of traditional panchakarma at home without the health risk often associated with in-clinic traditional panchakarma. To make this process even easier for you, we have put together in one single basket all the SVA Herbal Products you will need for Home PK – everything, start to finish. http://www.chandika.com/sva-7-week-home-pk-detox-basket/

AYURVEDIC MASSAGE (ABYHANGA)

Ayurvedic massage offers many benefits. If done in the morning, it helps you to start your day off relaxed, which is essential in maintaining balance.

When done at night, it promotes a restful night's sleep. It doesn't matter when you choose to do the massage, but you will receive the optimum benefits if you do it every day. Since the quality of Vata is dry and cold, a warm and oily massage provides an ideal balance for Vata types, though all types will notice increased health and vitality, especially during Vata season. The massage soothes the nervous system and the endocrine system, since skin produces endocrine hormones. It moisturizes and rejuvenates the skin, promoting a youthful appearance. It also helps the skin to eliminate toxins and tones the muscles.

It is possible to Abhyanga after your steam shower. Just make sure you apply only a thin layer of oil, not a thick one. Although the massage oils are rich in nutrients that nourish the physiology, they are also a detoxifying medium. By definition, oils pull out toxins, they bind the fat soluble toxins through the skin and pull them out of the cellular system. This is why Ayurveda recommends that we wait 20 minutes before washing off the oil, allowing time for the body to detox and the cellular system to be nourished. Since the SV Ayurveda oils have additional nutritional content, you may apply and leave the oil on after your shower for optimal absorption. At this time your channels will be open and even more receptive to all the transdermal nutrients. But make sure you apply a very thin layer, and not soak yourself in oil. Also, make sure that you wear warm clothes after applying the oil, because the oil molecules retain their temperature for a long time.

SV Ayurveda makes many wonderful specialty oils infused with herbs, vitamins and minerals. The Turmeric and Magnesium Massage Oil can be used by anyone. The Men's Rasayana Oil is made for men and the Women's Rasayana Oil is made especially for women. There are also oils to address the particular needs or your dosha. The Organic Coconut Oil is perfect for those hot summer months because it is cooling. The entire Abhyanga massage requires only about 2 ounces of oil each time.

http://www.chandika.com/body-massage-oils/-

Before you begin, warm the oil to skin temperature. The easiest way to do this is to keep a small plastic squeeze bottle filled with oil, and set the bottle in a bowl or cup of very hot water. Wait a few minutes for the oil to reach skin temperature.

- While the oil warms, lay out a towel to protect the carpet or floor from any oil that may spill.

- When you are ready, start the massage at your head. Drizzle a small amount of oil onto your scalp and massage it in with the palms of your hands. (You can skip the scalp part of the massage on days that you are not washing your hair.) Use a clockwise, circular motion. Then gently massage your face and ears. If you have oily skin, avoid those areas that are prone to breakouts. Massaging the ears is excellent for balancing Vata.

- Drizzle some oil in your palms and massage your neck, then move to your shoulders. Use a circular motion on your joints - shoulders, elbows, knees - and long up-and-down strokes on your limbs.

- Be gentle on your torso. Use large, clockwise motions to massage the chest and stomach area.

- Reach around to massage your back as best you can without straining.

- Then massage the legs, ankles, and knees. Using the palm of your hands, vigorously massage the feet.

- It is best to leave the oil on the body for 20 minutes before washing it off in a warm, not hot, shower or bath. You can use this time to meditate or do your Yoga exercises. If you don't have time to wait, that's fine. It's much better to do a quick massage than none at all.

The SVA massage oils undergo pranic prepping and special preservation methods that stop oxidization without compromising the intelligence of the oil base or the herbal infusions. With unique SVA formulations, you can now safely supplement your body with Magnesium, Vit D, Turmeric, and many more unique herbal and floral synergies. The benefits are innumerable:

- it transdermally nourishes the body with minerals and nutrients – depending on the oil you are using;

- pacifies all the doshas;

  relieves fatigue;

- provides stamina, and induces deep restful sleep at night;

- enhances the complexion and the luster of the skin;

- promotes longevity;
- Improves circulation;
- Gives mental clarity
- Increases Longevity
- Decreases the effects of aging
- Reduces Stress
- Strengthens Immune system
- Rejuvenates skin to make it smooth and support fat metabolism
- Softens and moisturizes the skin
- Lubricates the joints
- Calms the nerves
- Tones the muscles

Marma Point Self Massage

One of the most common ways that people gain excess weight is by emotional eating. When we feel stressed out over a period of time, for whatever reason, our emotions get the best of us and we tend to head for that comfort food. Have you ever noticed in the movies when someone gets their heart broken they take a big spoon and eat ice cream right out of the container? That's art, imitating life! Maybe this is the pattern we grew up with, such as Mom comforting us with a cookie when we got a 'boo-boo.' But there is also a scientific reason behind this phenomenon as well.

Any persistent stress on the mind or body causes the adrenal glands to release the hormone called cortisol. Cortisol increases appetite. The brain gets the signal that it needs more fuel to gather the strength to handle the stress. So we eat. When our digestive fire, or agni, is low, we don't metabolize what we're eating. The brain is confused, and asks: "Where are my nutrients?" so the appetite increases and then we overeat. And then all this food isn't metabolized properly so the channels get narrowed and ama accumulates, causing inflammation.

Unfortunately, stress seems to affect the foods we prefer. We're not bingeing on vegetables, we're craving foods high in fat and/or sugar. According to an study published in the Harvard Mental Health Newsletter, once ingested, these fatty and sugary foods have a feedback effect that "inhibits activity in the parts of the brain that produce and process stress and related emotions." Basically, even though we think these foods are helping us to relieve stress, they actually contribute to our stress-induced craving for fat and sugar. It's a vicious cycle.

Staying on our daily Ayurvedic routine definitely helps us to respond to stressors in a more healthy way. There are many studies showing that meditation reduces stress. Meditation also makes us more aware, so that we make better food choices. Exercise is another good tool to help us cope with stress. Some exercises, such as yoga and tai chi, combine both exercise and meditation. Social support also has a buffering effect on the way we experience stress. We need balance in our lives, and time with our family and friends, in person face to face, helps us to feel connected.

Ayurveda has given us another wonderful tool that helps us handle stress: Marma Therapy. This simple self-massage focuses on certain strategic points along the channels, or nadis, of the body. We can do a Marma Self-Massage in the morning before Abhyanga to help us prepare to handle stress. Or we can do a Marma Self-Massage in the evening to help remove stress.

Marma translates as "energy point." There are a total of 107 points in one body (besides the spine). Marmas are specific points on the physiology where the physical and subtle bodies meet. They respond to the sense of touch. Vaidya Mishra calls the marma points "switches" that turn on (or off) the flow of universal intelligence in the body, and thus support or repress life. Through the marmas we can address different stresses and imbalances in the physiology on various levels: physical, emotional, mental, vibrational. The marma massage administers balancing energy on different levels simultaneously making it vary safe, powerful and effective. The purpose of marma massage is more than to just deal with stress, it is to balance ourselves in these various levels so that we can experience true bliss, the bliss that was always meant to be ours.

Ayurveda says that there are certain factors that block this bliss from us. Any of these could be defined as "stress:"

- Environmental disturbances that affect the body's health

- Improper circulation of Prana (life-force) within the body in the channels

- Unresolved past grief and trauma

- Mental distractions preventing the mind from settling down and going inwards

- Sensory distractions that interfere with the ability to go within

Ayurveda characterizes certain herbs and spices as "divine" because they create a balanced chemistry in the physiology attuning it for higher states of consciousness. When we are in this place of restful awareness, stress can't affect the body and cause it to degenerate. The opposite also holds true: when the body is chemically balanced, it is easier for us to experience higher states of consciousness. Vaidya Mishra has created a kit called the "Samadhi Set" that consists of three herbalized creams to apply to specific marma points to support and enhance the feeling of bliss. http://www.chandika.com/samadhi-set-transdermal/

To massage the SVA marma points:

• Lightly touch the marma point with your finger and turn clockwise (as if you were looking at your body from the outside) 7-21 times in circles slightly larger than the size of a quarter. This should take between 10-15 seconds. You don't need to press, keep the touch light. Then hold lightly for another 10-15 seconds.

• Rest with your eyes closed for a few minutes and breathe in gently and deeply.

These are the recommended marma points to massage to prevent stress, relieve stress, and help you to find that place of bliss:

KRIKATIKA: BASE OF SKULL MARMA POINT:

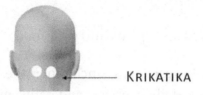

SHIRO GRIVA, BACK OF HEAD MARMA POINT

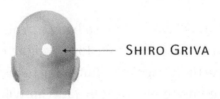

MANYA, COLLAR BONE MARMA POINT

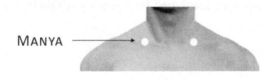

ANSA: MID-SHOULDER MARMA POINT

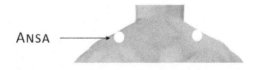

Summary

- For fat metabolism, this is the program:

- Eat easily digestible food

- Eat good fat

- Add herbs and spices into your food

- Follow Dinyacharya, including: the daily massages, daily exercise, and daily spiritual practice.

With this protocol, you will lose bad fat. You might not necessarily find that you lose weight on the scale, because this program is not going to just burn the fat, it is going to purify your fat. You will build up bone. You will lose clothing sizes. And you will have more energy and feel more radiant!

CHAPTER 3
Metabolize Your Sugar!

Sugar comes in all different forms. Glucose is the simplest form of sugar and is the sugar in blood, the body's primary source of energy. The white sugar we are familiar with is 99.9% sucrose. This sugar is refined from the natural sugar in sugar cane, with all the mineral ash and polyphenols removed. There are other forms of white sugar, such as baking sugar, powdered sugar, raw sugar, and they are all virtually identical to white sugar.

"Evaporated Cane Juice" is also sugar, with a bit lower sucrose content, so it tastes a little less sweet.

Brown sugar is 95% sucrose and 5% molasses. There are no nutritional benefits of brown sugar over white sugar.

Fructose, maltose, and dextrose are sugars that come from fruits and starchy plants. Lactose is the sugar that comes from dairy products. You can see the pattern that words that end with "ose" are all types of sugars. It is important to read packaging and labels when choosing foods, because sugars are in just about everything we eat. And there are often "hidden" sugars in food, so you need to be aware of what you are eating.

High fructose corn syrup (HFCS) is the main sweetener in most sodas and other carbonated beverages. HFCS is made with a chemical process and health experts are concerned about the level of genetic modification, environmental pollution and toxic processing used to create it. Basically, HFCS is not good for you, so stay away from it.

Agave syrup is a sugar substitute that comes from the Agave plant, a member of the cactus family. It is very high in fructose, as much as 92% fructose, depending on the brand. This is more than the body was meant to handle. Agave is not naturally sweet, it is processed, so it doesn't include many of the enzymes or nutrients that are in the original plant. In addition to this, Ayurveda says that the energy of the cactus is very harsh, so the energy of Agave is rajasic. Avoid using Agave as a sweetener.

Honey is a mix of sugars with other compounds, mostly fructose and glucose. It contains small amounts of vitamins and minerals and timy amount of antioxidants and anti-microbials. Honey differs in taste and composition depending on the flowers available to the bees that produce it. We need to be careful when selecting honey that the flowers used by the bees were not sprayed with pesticides, because those poisons get into the honey. Raw honey has not been processed, or has been minimally processed, so it may contain some pollen or small particles of wax from the hive.

When we see "sugar free" marked on packages it usually means that they include some sort of a sugar substitute, or sugar alcohol. Xylitol, Erythritol, Mannitol, Sorbitol and Glycerol are all examples of sugar alcohols. You'll see these listed as ingredients in sugar free candy for example. Notice the words all end in "ol." Sugar alcohols occur naturally in plants (including corn, so be careful if you have a corn allergy), but to extract them they must go through a highly-intensive industrial manufacturing process. These sugar substitutes are never fully absorbed but the body, so they can ferment in the intestines, causing gloating, gas, or diarrhea.

The sweeteners we find in restaurants in the little blue, pink or yellow packets are Saccharin Aspartame and Sucralose. If you read all the tiny print you'll find a "warning" on the package somewhere. All of these sugar substitutes are completely artificial and filled with chemicals.

While none have any calories or glycemic index, they have all been linked to digestive distress and chronic illnesses, including cancer, in research studies. Do not use these sweeteners at all!

Stevia is a South American herb that has been used as a sweetener for hundreds of years. It comes from the Stevia plant, and has a taste that can be 30 times sweeter than white sugar, and yet it doesn't have any calories. Stevia sweetener is made by crushing or distilling the leaves to form a powder or syrup. This gives it an intensely sweet flavor. Once stevia is refined like this it is even more sweet, so we only need to use a small amount. Stevia can have a bitter aftertaste that some people do not like. Vaidya Mishra has a range of natural sweeteners made from Stevia that he calls "Nectars." These Nectars are easily digestible with no aftertaste.

http://www.chandika.com/sva-sweet-nectar/

The main thing to remember about all these sugars is that what is important in Ayurveda is the taste. Even though the substitutes may have fewer calories, the result to the body is the same. The sweet taste confuses the body. Having the taste of sweet, no matter where that sweet comes from, notifies the brain that you are eating sweet. The brain sends the signal to the pancreas to make insulin. So this is a side effect of using sugar substitutes.

If you are already eating a food that is classified as "sweet" in Ayurveda, such as milk or rice pudding, then the result is not so bad. But adding any kind of sugar or "sweet" taste to a low glycemic food is going to give the pancreas that signal to create insulin anyway.

Scientifically, the glycemic index provides numerical values to help determine how quickly a food can raise blood sugar levels. This chart shows how foods rank, so you have more information when making choices as to which foods to favor and which to avoid. The higher the glycemic index number, the faster it raises blood sugar levels.

Ranking the glycemic index of foods

Foods that are considered "Low-GI Foods" have a glycemic index of 55 or less. These foods cause blood sugar to rise slowly, controlling insulin resistance. Low-GI foods also improve cholesterol levels, helping us to lose weight.

"Medium GI Foods" have a value between 56 and 69.

Any food with a value of 70 or more is considered a "High-GI Food." These foods raise blood sugar levels quickly. Most white foods are included on this list, as well as processed foods and foods made with white flour and white sugar.

Here are the numbers for some of the most common foods we eat:

Food Group	Food	Glycemic Index	Serving Size
Vegetables	Spinach	0	30g (1 cup)
	Green Beans	0	135g (1 cup)
	Cauliflower	0	100g (1 cup)
	Celery, raw	0	62g (1 stalk)
	Cabbage, cooked	0	75g (1/2 cup)
	Broccoli, cooked	0	78g (1/2 cup)
	Yams	51	136g (1 cup)
	Sweet Potatoes	54	133g (1 cup)
	Yellow Corn	55	166g (1 cup)
	Potato	104	213g (medium)
	Potato, baked	111	150g
	Potato, boiled	82	150g
	Parsnips	97	78g (1/2 cup)

Fruits	Sweet Cherries, raw	22	117g (1 cup)
	Plum	24	66g (1 fruit)
	Grapefruit	25	123g (1/2 fruit)
	Peach	28	98g (medium)
	Prunes	29	132g (1 cup)
	Dried Apricots	32	130g (1 cup)
	Pear	33	166g (medium)
	Apple, with skin	39	138g (medium)
	Strawberries	40	152g (1 cup)
	Grapes	43	92g (1 cup)
	Orange	48	140g (1 fruit)
	Banana	51	118g (medium)
	Mangos	51	165g (1 cup)
	Kiwi, with skin	58	76g (1 fruit)
	Papayas	60	140g (1 cup)
	Raisins	64	43g (small box)
	Cantaloupe	65	177g (1 cup)
	Pineapple	66	155g (1 cup)
	Watermelon	72	152g (1 cup)
Legumes	Peanuts	13	146g (1 cup)
	Soy Beans	20	172 (1 cup)
	Kidney Beans	27	256g (1 cup)
	Lentils	29	198g (1 cup)

	Chickpeas, boiled	31	240g (1 cup)
	Pinto Beans	39	171g (1 cup)
	Lima Beans	31	241g (1 cup)
	Baked Beans	48	254g (1 cup)
Nuts	Cashews	22	N/A
	Hazelnuts	0	N/A
	Almonds	0	N/A
	Macadamia Nuts	0	N/A
	Pecans	0	N/A
	Walnuts	0	N/A
Beverages	Whole Milk	40	244g (1 cup)
	Plain Yogurt	36	245g (1 cup)
	Tomato Juice	38	243g (1 cup)
	Apple Juice	41	248g (1 cup)
	Soy Milk	44	245g (1 cup)
	Grapefruit Juice	48	250g (1 cup)
	Orange Juice	57	249g (1 cup)

Grains	Quinoa	53	150g (1 cup)
	White Rice	89	150g (1 cup)
	Brown Rice	50	150g (1 cup)
	Bulgur	48	150g (1 cup)
	Couscous	65	150g (1 cup)
	Pearled Barley	28	150g (1 cup)
Cereals	Oatmeal	55	250g (1 cup)
	Bran Cereal	55	30g (1 cup)
	Puffed Wheat	80	30g (1 cup)
Breads	Kaiser Roll	73	57g (1 roll)
	Bagel	72	89g (1/4 in.)
	Glazed donut	76	75g (large)
	White Bread	70	25g (1 slice)
	Wheat Bread	70	28g (1 slice)
	Pita bread, white	68	30g
	Corn tortilla	52	50g
	Wheat tortilla	30	50g
Other	Hummus	6	30g
	Popcorn	55	8g (1 cup)

As you can see, some foods that are generally considered healthy, and good for us, have a high glycemic index. So if we have any issue with sugar metabolism, they are *not* good for us.

From an Ayurvedic perspective, even though the western medical industry has given milk a low-medium glycemic index, we have not found this to be true. It may be the milk industry lobby or some other reason that this number is artificially low. Vaidya Mishra has found that his patients who have problems with glucose metabolism have huge sugar spikes after consuming milk. So SV Ayurveda recommends avoiding milk altogether. Instead substitute with almond milk, or the 20% yogurt mixed with 80% water beverage.

Foods Supporting Sugar Metabolism

When you have high blood sugar levels, it is of course a medical condition and you should work with your medical doctor to address it. However, even a traditional western medical doctor will recommend that you reduce or eliminate foods that have a high sugar content.

You need to do two things to help your body to better metabolize sugar. Number one: you need to see why it has gotten to that point, what has caused it, and try to address and correct the cause. Number two: you need to stop putting high sugar content foods into your body, since your body is already unable to process and digest the sugar. These two things help you to maintain optimal levels of blood sugar. In terms of diet, this helps those who already are struggling with a diabetic condition by giving them informed choices. But this program is also for those who want a healthier, less-sugar containing diet for any other personal, non-medical reasons.

However, the energy and nourishment that we get from glucose is necessary. That is why we crave it. Some glucose in your diet is necessary. That's why it is essential NOT to completely eliminate ALL sugar containing food items (grains, lentils, fruits, etc), but to choose correctly the foods that have less, rather than more, glycemic indices or content. It is also important to learn how to cook foods properly – how much cooking, in what method, and with what spices. The trick is to make your food easily digestible so that your stomach can digest it faster, your colon can absorb it faster, and the liver and the pancreas can transform the sugar into energy fully and more quickly.

If you have a tendency towards having low blood sugar levels, hypoglycemia, then you should follow the recommendations in this program with caution. You should probably supplement your diet with some higher GI foods and fruits so that your levels don't drop too low.

Are You Spice Deficient?

There is much talk about getting the required vitamins and minerals we need – and fear of becoming "deficient" in any essential nutrients. However, not much is said about the spice deficiency that is prevalent today. Ayurveda is very clear that food is our best medicine, and spices are foods that we need to help the body function efficiently. How do you recognize if you are spice deficient? First understand all that spices can do for the body. Here are some of the symptoms that pop up when you are lacking spice in your diet:

- **Indigestion**. Spices help support the digestion. If you have too much acid present in the body, you need cooling, calming, alkalizing spices.

- **Bowel issues**. Ayurveda says we need a balance between digestion, absorption and elimination, and spices help this to happen. Whether you are constipated or have diarrhea herbs can help.

- **Fatigue**. Most people report that they feel fatigued after lunch, but this is not the way it is supposed to be. If you do not want to be tired after a meal, use spices in your food to open the channels and create oxidization to the system. Some people feel tired after eating sweets. But add some spice to the sweet and there's no drowsiness.

- Lack of energy and enthusiasm. This is a sign of spice deficiency. There's a reason for the saying "variety is the spice of life!" Spice up your life when you spice up your foods and you will feel the difference with a boost in your levels of energy and enthusiasm.

Interestingly, when certain spices are added to foods it lowers the glycemic index of that food. This is because in the cooking process there is a molecular interaction and the sugar becomes more mild, and easier to digest. So it is always a good idea to cook with spices. The best spices to support digestion and sugar metabolism are: fenugreek, cinnamon, ginger, turmeric and black pepper.

When we cook lentils, for example, with these spices the glycemic index is lowered by about 10 points. The same thing happens with any kind of rice. Cook rice with these spices and you will lower the glycemic index of the rice. All of the spices mentioned above are good, but cinnamon is the best spice to use for this purpose. The caveat is that we should not eat too much of any one spice – it is always best to combine spices.

We often find spices like cinnamon and fenugreek sold in capsule form in grocery or health food stores, but this is not a good way to get spices into our system. Always cook with spices so that you get the molecular interaction with food and the spices make their way into your system slowly. We can also add spices to salads, especially salads made with cucumber. White or dark radish has a low glycemic index and it also helps to eliminate toxins. Romaine lettuce is very good in a salad. We can make salad dressings with yogurt and add spice to it as well.

Many good fruits have a very high glycemic index: mango, watermelon, or oranges for example – so we need to be careful about eating too much fruit. However, when you crave something like a fresh apple or pear, you can slice them and sprinkle some cumin seed, soma salt, lime juice, or Mom's masala on the slices and that will lower the glycemic index.

While western medicine looks only at the glycemic index number of a food for sugar metabolism, SV Ayurveda also looks at the properties of the food in terms of how it functions in your channels. For example, green peas and soy have a low glycemic index, so a western nutritionist might recommend these foods. But SV Ayurveda knows that both green peas and soy are very bad for your channels so Vaidya Mishra does not recommend them.

A western nutritionist might recommend eating bananas, noting that they are high in nutrients like potassium. But they haven't learned about the ultimate effect that the banana molecules have of clogging the physical channels. Western medicine doesn't have this system of studying the ingredients in place.

Western nutritionists often recommend eating lima beans and pinto beans because they have a lower glycemic index and they are also high in protein. But western medicine doesn't understand that if you do not digest food 100%, that any percent you don't digest becomes semi-digested material, or Ama, and that Ama is the seed of millions of diseases.

But now you know this! And you can make more informed decisions on your own as to which foods you want to eat for your optimal health.

Ingredients That Support Sugar Metabolism

- **Spices**: Cinnamon, cinnamon leaf, fenugreek, turmeric, black pepper, cumin, coriander, clove, green cardamom, black cardamom

- **Grains**: barley, rye, organic whole what, basmati rice cooked with spices

- **Fats**: ghee, sesame oil, olive oil

- **Lentils** (Dahl): kala chana, mung, massoor

- **Vegetables**: karela, dark bitter leafy greens, Brussels sprouts, methi leaf

- **Sweeteners**: honey, fructose

- **Dairy**: lassi (yogurt and water blend)

- **Fruit**: apple, cherry, grapefruit, pear, prunes, apricot

- **Meat**: white meat (if you eat meat protein)

Bitter melon is actually a vegetable, also known as "karela" or bitter gourd, is very good for sugar metabolism. The reason is that it is bitter, just as the name implies. There are two kinds of bitter melon, one is Chinese and the other is Indian.

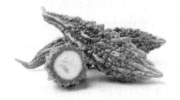

Karela - Bitter Melon

Be sure to buy the Indian variety because that one is truly bitter in taste. The bitter taste helps to purify the liver and the pancreas. Bitter leafy greens are also good for sugar metabolism, but too much of them can clot your blood because they contain a lot of vitamin K. If you are on blood thinners then bitter leafy greens are contraindicated. However baby spinach or tender leafy greens are very good. But karela is really one of the best overall foods for sugar metabolism. Vaidya Mishra says that his patients who eat karela every day see their glucose levels decrease.

Methi leaves come from the fenugreek plant. They are too bitter to eat on their own, so mix them with some thyme, and use this half and half with other greens. This is very good simply stir-fried in sesame oil with some cumin and Mom's masala, and just a little bit of Soma Salt.

It is important to remember that to really support your glucose system, do not let yourself get too hungry. When you start to feel hungry, eat something low glycemic. Don't starve yourself and let your blood sugar levels dip. Maintain a healthy blood sugar level rather than allowing your levels to spike and plummet. When you follow the Ayurvedic routine, Dinyacharya, you'll be eating at the same time each day and your levels will be steady.

Just as exercise is essential for fat metabolism, it is also essential for glucose metabolism. Exercise has to be a part of our daily routine.

Herbs Supporting Sugar Metabolism

Gymnema has been getting a lot of publicity recently as a super-herb to metabolize sugar and also supporting the body's ability to produce insulin. Gymnema is also called gurmar, or sugar-killer. Gymnema does not taste bitter at all, but it totally diffuses the sweet power of sugar molecules right away. If you take some gymnema, either by chewing it or drinking it in a brew, and then eat sugar within five minutes, the sugar will have no taste at all. There will be no sweetness there for you to be able to identify it as sugar – you might think it is sand!

Vaidya Mishra has created a whole line of oral care products where the main ingredient is gymnema. When you brush your teeth with this toothpaste, or spray the oral mist in your mouth, all the sugar molecules get diffused, and there is no food for the bad bacteria to feed on in your mouth. So the bad bacteria starve and die, and your mouth remains fresh for hours!

If you have a tendency towards low blood sugar then you will not want to use gymnema as it lowers your blood sugar levels.

Another herb that lowers glucose levels is Indian kino. It comes from a huge tree called Vijayasar. In India they make a cup from the wood of the tree that you drink from to lower sugar levels. Indian kino does not taste bitter, but it does taste astringent, which is also good for glucose reduction. Researchers have found that there is a specific cell in the pancreas called the "lingering cell" and Indian kino helps to regenerate this cell. It is a very powerful herb, very supportive to the pancreas.

There is a fruit in India called jamun. The English name for it is black plum. Jamun is very sweet, and when it is ripe it becomes black. The seed of the jamun is especially cooling for the pancreas. The pancreas is a very dense organ, as is the liver. When the pancreas is hot, is creates less insulin, and insulin that is less pure. SV Ayurveda says that the cooling properties of jamun seed help the pancreas very much. You can use jamun seed to support glucose metabolism. However, if you have a medical condition, check with your doctor before using jamun seed. If you are on anti-diabetic insulin or any medication, this can be too much for your system and you could go into hypoglycemia.

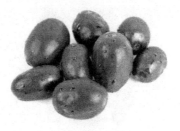

Jamun – Indian Black Plum

Ayurveda has many more recommended herbs to support glucose metabolism. These are just a few that you can use easily in your daily life. Vaidya Mishra has made it easy for us with his new coffee substitute that contains gymnema, Indian kino, and jamun seed. It is a coffee substitute because it has no coffee, and no caffeine, and yet it smells and tastes just like espresso. And it give you energy like espresso does as well! The energy comes from using your own glucose that goes to your muscles, nerves and brain after having this coffee substitute. It is best to drink this after a meal so you have some starch and glucose to metabolize with the gymnema brew.

http://www.chandika.com/gymnema-brew/

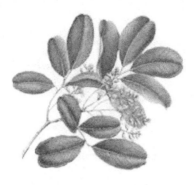

Indian Kino

Herbs That Support Sugar Metabolism

- **Gymnema**: Gymnema Sylvestre
  http://www.chandika.com/gymnema-leaf/

- **Indian Kino**: Pterecarpus Marsupium
  http://www.chandika.com/indian-kino-herbal-memory-nectar/

- **Jamun Seed**: Syzygium Cumini
  http://www.chandika.com/jamun-seeds/

- **Neem**: Azadirachta Indica
  http://www.chandika.com/neem-leaf/

CHAPTER 4
The Art of Eating for Optimal Digestion

There's a reason why mom always told us to sit up straight at the table, and to chew with our mouths closed. Yes, she wanted us to learn good manners, and she probably also wanted us to digest our food properly. Ayurveda has very simple guidelines that we can follow to make sure that the digestion system can function most efficiently.

-It's always nice to set the table for a meal. Remove clutter and provide a calm atmosphere in which to eat. From the moment we sit down the body begins to anticipate a meal, and starts preparing itself for digestion.

-Eat only when you are hungry. And eat before you get so hungry that you are uncomfortable. 3-5 hours between meals is usually best.

-Stop eating when you feel about 50-75% full. Don't overstuff yourself. Eating too much food overloads your digestive system and can lead to a build-up of toxins. Ayurveda calls these toxins "ama" – it's a sticky waste product of digestion that clogs the channels of circulation in the body so that nutrients can't get to where they need to go. Ama in the body makes us feel heavy and dull. And over time, if we don't get rid of the ama, we may experience constipation or diarrhea, joint pain, or even a lowered immune system.

-Sit down while eating, and pay attention to the meal that you are eating. When we stand there's a part of our brain that stays in "fight or flight" mode, ready to go. When we sit we are more relaxed. Take this time to really taste the food, smell the food, take in the colors of the food. This helps to make the experience of eating more pleasant.

-Don't watch TV or read while you are eating. And don't talk on the phone or drive while eating. All of these activities just serve as a distraction to the food that interrupts the digestive process and can cause you to overeat. Connect your mind with your food. When you focus on your food, and pay attention to the tastes, colors and smells, your body and mind will be able to work more efficiently to digest the food properly.

-Make sure to include all six tastes (sweet, sour, salty, bitter, pungent, and astringent) in each meal so that you feel satisfied after you eat. Most of the time when we get those cravings after dinner, when we feel like we need "more" or we want to go back for second helpings, it's because we are lacking one or more of those six tastes. Including all of the six tastes keeps us satiated so that the meal itself is enough for us.

-Avoid ice-cold food and beverages. Cold water douses the digestive fire. At a restaurant, ask for water without ice. Adding a slice of lemon is also beneficial in stimulating digestion. Lemon is warming, which is balancing for Vatas and Kaphas. Lime is cooling, which is better for Pittas, and better for all of us during the hot summer months.

-Sit quietly for a few minutes after eating. Don't rush to your next activity. Spend some time being still and grateful for the meal.

It may take a little getting used to these new good habits, but you'll see the difference it makes in your digestion, and your energy level, very quickly. This way of eating is something we all need to pass on to our children and families. No more eating standing up over the kitchen sink!

CHAPTER 5

The Importance of Protein

In the ayurvedic understanding, our tissues are built one of top of the other; one tissue nourishes the next. The muscle tissue nourishes the fat tissue. This means that if your muscle tissue is healthy and happy, it will supply the needed nutrients to your fat tissue. Protein is food for the muscle tissue, or mamsa dhatu.

Ayurveda recommends a plant-based diet - vegetarian rather than vegan. SV Ayurveda says to avoid processed cheeses, and to choose paneer, preferably home-made paneer. Instead of butter, choose yogurt-based ghee, and instead of dairy milk, choose almond milk. These choices also provide needed calcium to the diet.

Vegans need to be careful to get enough calcium in their diets since they are not eating dairy foods. Fortunately there are many foods that provide good calcium so that we don't need to resort to some of the not-good-for-us sources of calcium, such as the calcium in many over-the-counter supplements that include grounded bone. When we eat "bad" calcium, or when the body can't process good calcium, or when the metabolic power of the bone tissue isn't good, then you get microcalcification. Microcalicification can occur in any part of the body. It narrows the channels and affects fat metabolism negatively. Fat accumulation can create bone calcification, making you susceptible to kidney stones.

If you are looking for a calcium supplement, Soma-Cal Capsules from SV Ayurveda

http://www.chandika.com/soma-cal-capsules/

contain "good" calcium, from the branch of the coral, not the root, so it is soft and easy to assimilate. In the Ayurvedic texts it says that the molecule of "prawal" or the soft part of coral, is as healthy as the calcium found in mother's milk.

In our tissue system, the fat tissue comes before the bone tissue. When the fat does not transform to bone, it accumulates and then we gain weight.

Kulti is a lentil that is high in protein and minerals, including calcium. It is a powerful, intelligent lentil that has the power to disintegrate the micromolecules of calcification and it can even help break up kidney stones. SV Ayurveda makes an instant protein powder with kulti and barley that has a low glycemic index. Barley is an ingredient famous in Ayurveda for its weight loss properties.

For some people who are vegan, or who are transitioning to a plant-based diet after having had animal protein in their diet for many years, they may struggle with finding a suitable protein source to provide the B12, Amino Acids, and/or Iron they require. The problem with many protein substitutes is that they are processed so much that the ingredients in them lose their natural intelligence. This natural intelligence is what allows the protein to become molecules that get delivered to the muscles, neurotransmitters, and wherever they need to go in the body to do their job. Vaidya Mishra has created a plant-based protein powder in such a way that the protein molecules are protected from oxidation when it is being prepared. And he found a way to protect these protein molecules from oxidation so that they don't lose their intelligence when they go through protein synthesis. You can use the ***SVA Instant Tridoshic Vegan Protein Powder***

http://www.chandika.com/vegan-protein-

powder in many ways, including adding it to juices.

Juicing is convenient, fast, and creates beverages packed with nutritionally high fresh ingredients. But is juicing really as healthy as it is made out to be? In ayurvedic terms, it depends on what's in the beverage, and also how and when you are consuming it. If we take it one step further, in SVA terms, we also consider this:

- The beverage should be rich and nourishing, but without suppressing or putting out your digestive fire.

- The beverage should be satiating, but not heavy and clogging so that it blocks your channels.

- The beverage should balance all your doshas, without aggravating or depleting any of them.

Unfortunately, the juicing gurus mix in ingredients without considering how the ingredients combine, or interact with each other, adding protein powders, dehydrated vegetable powders, soy, and all kinds of things. Long-term consumption will certainly confirm that such recipes cause more harm than good. Because so many of Vaidya Mishra's clients have asked about juicing with such enthusiasm, he created an ancient ayurvedic method of consuming a nourishing and refreshing protein shake on-the-go.

In India there is a practice of consuming dehydrated lentil powders, blended in with different spices, in addition to water, or yogurt, to rehydrate oneself in the high heat temperatures. Inspired by this ancient ayurvedic tradition, Vaidya Mishra came up with ***SVA Instant Tridoshic Vegan Protein Powder.***

http://www.chandika.com/vegan-protein-powder

This is a nutritious, easy-to-use powder with which you can make shakes or smoothies. You can even sprinkle on your cooked rice, salads, or soups. It primarily contains dry-roasted and pulverized kala chana (black chickpeas). In India, kala chana is a high-protein ingredient used in many delicious recipes.

Kala Chana is a variation of the commonly known larger variety of chickpea. It is smaller and darker in color, and high in protein. It carries a very low glycemic index and is a great source of protein for vegetarians who have sugar intolerance, or are diabetic.

To make our SVA Vegan Protein Shake Powder, Vaidya Mishra uses only black chickpeas and roasts them according to the traditional method used in India. After roasting, we remove the tough husk of the chickpeas, which can irritate the digestive track when consumed. Then we grind the roasted kala chana down to a fine powder. Roasting it this way makes the otherwise heavy chana light and easy to digest. This processing also keeps all the components of the raw food intact with no loss of any nutrient. SVA Vegan Protein Powder is not only tri-doshic, meaning balancing to all three doshas, it is also soy-free and gluten-free.

Nutritional Overview: Instant Vegan High-Protein SVA Shake

The main ingredients in the SVA Vegan Protein Powder, Kala chana, is a very famous ingredient in Ayurveda. It has been used traditionally to aid in the control of diabetes and chronic skin conditions. Not only is it a good source of protein, Kala chana also aids weight loss, cardiac health, and cleans the colon.

Kala chana is high in protein, and low in fat. Besides building and maintaining healthy muscles, protein is needed to synthesize hormones and neurotransmitters. Therefore, everyone can benefit from a quick supplement of high-quality protein in shake form.

If you are a vegan, you can use this powder even more liberally in addition to your shakes or smoothies. You can sprinkle the powder on your food to provide for any essential protein you may be missing from your diet.

Kala chana also provides high amounts of dietary fiber needed to help lower cholesterol, regulate blood sugar, and provide healthy intestinal flora and bowel movements. Kala chana is also rich in easy-to-absorb minerals and vitamins – especially iron, calcium, potassium and folate.

Other protein powders: One of the reasons that Vaidya Mishra decided to make this high protein powder was that so many of his clients were supplementing their protein intake with unhealthy alternatives, such as soy, green peas, and whey powders. These mixes are very popular in the marketplace, but aren't very good for you at all. Here's why:

The problem with soy: While it is true that soy beans provide a rich source of amino acids, it is equally true that all that glitters is not gold! In SVA, we know to look beyond the label to see a food's ultimate effect on the doshas, tissues, physical channels, and vibrational channels. Soy is a major 'channel blocker,' consumption of which is suitable only by those doing hard physical labor day in day out – not at all suitable for the diet of the office or professional worker. Soy is also highly estrogenic and can promote many disturbances in the female physiology. To avoid such problems and to keep your channels open, steer clear of soy-based protein supplements.

The problem with green peas: Peas and pea-based protein powders are *mahavistambhi*. Maha means 'great,' vistambhi means 'clogging' or 'blocking.' That is to say, peas are first-class channel blockers, even more so than soy. They will slow down your overall metabolic system, promote the production of toxins, or ama, and long-term cause many unwanted imbalances. For those who already experience joint pain or joint related conditions, green peas should be avoided.

Whey or No Way? Whey protein is a mixture of globular proteins isolated from whey, the liquid material created as a by-product of cheese production. Not only is whey clogging to the channels, it is also highly acidic. We know that the physiology needs a good pH level to be healthy. While eating whey provides protein, it also unnecessarily introduces more acidity into the physiology. In addition, as a protein isolate, whey has lost the intelligence originally found in its milk source and has become a 'dumb' protein. Dumb foods (those with less *prana*) are more difficult to digest and more likely to produce ama (toxins).

Delicious Instant Vegan High-Protein Shake Powder recipes

Your Instant Protein Powder is ready to eat. Almost. Even with all the processing, the liveliness of black chana is still there. However, with proper samyog (combination) and proper samskar (processing) the powder can be enjoyed by all constitutions and all types of agni – your body's digestive power: 1) vishmagni (variable); 2) tiksnagni (sharp); 3) mandagni (slow); and 4) samagni (balanced).

Vata (vishmagni)

Some people have variable appetite and digestion. If this sounds like you, then you are probably a Vata mind/body type, and this this recipe would be good for you. Blend well:

Spring water: 8 oz.
Instant Vegan Protein Powder: 2 TBSP
Raw sugar: ½ tsp.
Soma Salt: add per taste
Lime juice: 1 TBSP
Cumin seeds (dry roasted and ground): ¼ tsp.
Grated ginger (optional): ¼ tsp.
Green chili (optional): small piece

Pro-biotic variation: Same as above with 1 TBSP homemade, fresh yogurt. Blend in blender 3 – 5 minutes.

Pitta (high agni, high pitta)

Some people always have intense hunger and an intense appetite. If this sounds like you, you are probably a Pitta type with high agni (digestive fire). Try this recipe. Blend:

Spring water: 8 oz.
Instant Vegan Protein Powder: 4 TBSP
Rose Petal Preserve: 1 tsp. or rose powder ½ tsp.
Raw sugar: 1 tsp. (not needed if using rose preserve)

Pro-biotic variation: Same as above with 4 TBSP homemade, fresh yogurt. Blend in blender 3 – 5 minutes.

Pitta (low agni)

Those people with heat, acidity, along with poor digestion and less hunger are usually high in Pitta, but low in agni. This is the recipe for them: Blend in blender:

Spring water: 8 oz.
Instant Vegan Protein Powder: 2 TBSP
Fennel seeds (toasted and ground): ½ tsp
Rose Petal Preserve: 1/2 tsp. or rose powder 1/4 tsp.
Raw sugar: 1/2 tsp. (not needed if using rose preserve)
Clove: 1 bud
Green Cardamom: 1 pod

Pro-biotic variation: Same as above with 1 TBSP homemade, fresh yogurt. Blend in blender 3 – 5 minutes.

Kapha (mandagni)

This recipe is best for kapha constitutions and those with heavy, slow digestion and low appetite. Blend:

Spring water: 8 oz.
Instant Vegan Protein Powder: 2 TBSP
Black pepper ground: 1/8 tsp
Soma Salt: add per taste
Lime juice: 1 TBSP

Kapha Garcinia Masala: ½ tsp. First toast in 1 tsp. of Mom's Ghee

Pro-biotic variation: Same as above with 1 TBSP homemade, fresh yogurt. Blend in blender 3 – 5 minutes.

Fat metabolism and Weight loss recipe

Blend:

Spring water: 8 oz.
Instant Vegan Protein Powder: 4 TBSP
MedAgni Masala: ½ tsp
Soma Salt: add per taste
Lime juice: 1 TBSP

Pro-biotic variation: Same as above with 2 TBSP homemade, fresh yogurt. Blend in blender 3 – 5 minutes.

Muscle Gain Formula

If your muscle tissue needs more support and nourishment, boil milk and water together first. Blend:

Spring water: 4 oz.
Organic milk: 4 oz.
Instant Vegan High-Protein Shake Powder: 4 TBSP
Ghee: 1 tsp.
Rose Petal Preserve: 1/2 tsp.
Raw sugar: 1 tsp. (not needed if using rose preserve)
Green Cardamom: 1 pod

Sugar Metabolism Formula

This recipe will enhance sugar metabolism. Do not use if you have tendency to low blood sugars or hypoglycemia. Make the soup mix first by adding and mixing in just boiled water. After it cools to comfortable temperature add the mix and other ingredients. Blend well. Drink.

Spring water: 10 oz.
Instant Vegan High-Protein Shake Powder: 3 TBSP
Karela Soup Mix: 1 TBSP
Soma Salt: add by taste
Lime juice: 1 TBSP

Veggies and Protein

You can also enjoy SVA Vegan Protein Powder with cooked vegetables. Chop and boil a zucchini squash, add a few leafy greens (kale, swiss chard, etc) or a handful or two of baby spinach leaves, throw in a carrot, etc. Then add your vegetables to your mixture of Protein Powder, in addition to a 1/4 tsp Mom's Masala, some olive oil, Soma Salt to taste, and a squirt of lime. Blend and enjoy!

Green-Protein

Use any kind or combination of leafy greens that you like: baby spinach leaves, collard greens, Swiss chard, dinosaur or purple kale. Steer away from mustard greens as they tend to be a little heating and pitta aggravating.

80% by weight leafy greens
20% by weight fresh cheese (paneer)
A few sprigs of Italian Parsley (flat preferred but curly is fine)
¼ cup spring water
½ teaspoon Mom's Masala
½ teaspoon Mom's Ghee
¼ teaspoon Soma Salt
Fresh Thai Chili (optional)
Fresh Ginger – 2 slices (optional)
¼ teaspoon Olive oil

Use a large fry pan or skillet. Add ghee to the pan, along with the Mom's Masala (and chili and ginger if you are using these). Add the paneer chunks and sauté for a couple of minutes.

Remove most of the stems from the greens. Chop the greens and parsley all together and add to the pan with the paneer. Add the water.

Cover the top and cook for only as long as it takes to allow the greens to turn bright green in color.

Remove from pan and put everything in the blender.

Add water as needed and blend to a perfect smooth texture. Hot water is recommended by room temperature is fine, too.

When ready to serve, squirt some fresh lime on top and stir it in. Enjoy!

CHAPTER 6
Recipes

Paneer

Home-made Indian Cheese

Use fresh, raw milk. Make just as much paneer as you need at a time.

In a heavy-bottomed pot bring milk to a boil.
Add enough fresh-squeezed lime juice (Approx. 1 lime per half gallon of milk) to curd/yogurt
Milk curdles into white solids and clear green liquid (whey)
Strain through cheesecloth.
Discard the whey.
For firmer cheese, place weight on top or hang the cheesecloth from a hook for an hour or so to strain out more liquid.

Short cut: You can also strain using a fine mesh strainer instead of cheesecloth. Press the paneer with a spoon to remove the excess liquid.

Home-made Yogurt SVA Style

It's so nice to make fresh yogurt daily right in your own kitchen. And it's so easy to do there's no reason not to. You control the ingredients, you know exactly what you are putting into the yogurt and into your body. If you want it to be super-easy, you can get a yogurt-making machine. Just don't leave the yogurt in the machine too long or it will get too sour. 3 hours is a good amount of time.

Without a machine, here's the recipe:

Start with organic raw milk. Raw milk is non-homogenized, so it is more pure. For every 1 quart of milk, use 2-3 Tablespoons of already-made yogurt as a starter. For your first batch use a yogurt from the store, select a high-quality, organic, plain yogurt.

Heat the milk in a saucepan on medium on the stove. When the milk foams up, turn off the heat and let it cool to body temperature, or around 100 degrees Fahrenheit if you are using a thermometer.

Meanwhile, let the already-made yogurt that you are using come to room temperature. You don't want to add cold yogurt to the warm milk.

Pour the warm milk into a large jar. Mix in the yogurt.

Cover the jar and put the jar in a warm, draft free place. The inside of your oven with the light on works well. Leave it there for 6-8 hours. Then it will be ready and you can refrigerate it.

Remember to save out some yogurt for your next batch!

SVA Spiced Yogurt

8 oz of water – room temperature
2 oz yogurt
Soma salt to taste
Mom's Masala, 4 pinches
Blend together
Optional: add finely chopped Green Chilies

Karela (Bitter Melon)

1 serving
Karela, 8 oz chopped thin
Turmeric, ½ teaspoon
Coriander, 1 teaspoon toasted and ground
Soma Salt to taste
Cumin Seed, ¼ teaspoon
Sweet Tamarind, 2 oz
Grated Ginger, ½ teaspoon
Ghee or Sesame Oil, 1 teaspoon
Curry leaf (optional) 4 leaves
Green Chili (optional) 1

- Toast lightly in ghee of sesame oil: turmeric, cumin, chili, and grated ginger. Be careful not to burn the spices.
- Add think pieces of Karela with Soma Salt and tamarind paste.
- Cover and cook over low to medium flame for 15 minutes.
- Add toasted coriander powder and cook five more minutes.

Karela is usually very bitter in taste. Coriander and sweet tamarind remove the bitterness, while the spices lend extra delicious flavor to this dish.

SVA Karela Instant Soup

Karela Instant Soup Mix – SVA Proprietary Blend

Ingredients:
Karela (high potency freeze-dried)
Coriander Seed
Cumin Seed
Arrowroot Powder

- Mix well 1 Tablespoon of soup mix in 8 oz of cool water
- Boil five minutes covered. Remove from heat.
- Add Soma Salt to taste, a few drops of olive oil, a few drops of fresh lime juice, and garnish with chopped cilantro.

Karela Instant Soup mix is delicious eaten as is. For even greater enjoyment, you can add your favorite cooked vegetables to your soup.

Tip: The ideal temperature for cooking is medium heat. When you cover the pot you don't need a high temperature because steam cooks the food nicely. Slower cooking is better to bring out the best in foods.

Kala Chana Dahl

1 serving

Kala chana dahl, 4 oz
Organic turmeric powder, ¼ teaspoon
Soma Salt to taste
Garcinia Masala, ½ teaspoon (Vata, Pitta, or Kapha)
OR Mango Powder, ½ teaspoon
MedAgni Masala, ¼ teaspoon
Mom's Ghee, 1 teaspoon
Cumin, ¼ teaspoon
Green Chili (optional), ½

- Boil dahl with turmeric in 16 oz of spring water in a covered pot until soft (approx.. 20-25 minutes)

- In a separate pan, lightly toast the cumin, garcinia (or mango powder), MedAgni Masala, and chili (optional) in Mom's Ghee.

- Stir the ghee mixture into the dahl and let set for a minute or two.

-Sprinkle fresh lime juice over top just before serving.

Chana has the lowest glycemic index of any dahl. Chana alone is difficult to digest. This cooking process and these ingredients make chana digestible and flavorful. Chana Dahl helps to synthesize protein molecules and supports both fat and sugar metabolism. It goes great with any grain. This dish is high in protein and fiber and has a low glycemic index.

Tip: If you soak the chana dahl for 6-8 hours before cooking it will cook more quickly. Soaking also makes the dahl more easily digestible.

MedAgni Masala is especially designed to support the fire that metabolizes fat. It is semi-toasted. You can cook with it or you can use it in the yogurt drink mix.

Basil Barley Spring Salad

1 serving

Barley pearls, 4 oz
Spring water, 8 oz
Mom's Ghee, 1 teaspoon
Sliced almonds, 1 Tablespoon
Fresh Basil, 1 teaspoon chopped
Soma Salt to taste
Fresh Lime juice
Virgin Olive Oil, cold pressed
Crushed Black Peppercorn, ¼ teaspoon

- Boil barley pearls until they break (approx.. 20 minutes)

- Lightly toast the sliced almonds in Mom's Ghee

- Add Soma Salt to taste.

- Spoon cooked barley into a serving dish, top with sliced almonds, black pepper and olive oil.

-Sprinkle lime juice over everything just before serving.

Tip: Always use lime juice, fresh squeezed on top of already cooked, don't cook the citrus juice. Lime is alkalizing, it don't make your body acidic. But when you cook this juice, it becomes acidic. The body cannot buffer the acid to neutralize it. When you sprinkle fresh lime juice you get all the benefits without creating any toxins or inflammation in the body.

Lime is good for so many things. It has ascorbic acid (Vitamin C), and many other antioxidants. Lemon is also good, but the buffering time is longer. Lime transforms alkalinity faster than lemon, so SV Ayurveda recommends lime.

Sesame Ginger Broccoli

1 serving

Organic broccoli, 1 cup of florets in chopped into bite-sized pieces
Sesame oil, 1 Tablespoon
Almonds, 2 Tablespoons chopped and blanched
Fresh Ginger, 1 teaspoon grated
Sesame Seeds, 1 Tablespoon
Soma Salt to Taste
Lime Juice
Green Chili (optional), 1

- Steam the broccoli until bright green. It should be tender but not soggy. Spoon into serving dish.

- Lightly toast the almonds, ginger and chili (optional) in the sesame oil. Drizzle over the broccoli and stir.

- Dry toast the sesame seeds lightly. Sprinkle over the broccoli.

-Add Soma Salt and a squeeze of fresh lime over everything.

Assorted Fruit Bowl

Kiwi – chopped in bite sized pieces
Blueberries
Cherries, pitted
Blackberries
Soma Salt
Mom's Spice Mix

- Put equal parts of each fruit in a bowl. Sprinkle Soma Salt and Mom's Masala over the assortment of fruit.

The assorted fruit bowl is a fantastic mid-afternoon pick-me-up. A low-glycemic treat great for when you need a little something to satisfy hunger between lunch and dinner.

Mom's Spice Mix, also known as Mom's Masala, is a unique and delicious combination of toasted spices that contains all six tastes so it is balancing for all the doshas.

http://www.chandika.com/sva-moms-masala/

Very Berry Seeds and Nuts

Fresh Berries (any kind or combination)
Sunflower seeds
Chopped Almonds
Soma Salt
Mom's Spice Mix
Spring Water
Lime Juice (optional)

- Soak the berries, almonds, and sunflower seeds all together overnight in spring water. Be careful not to use too much water.

- Strain any sunflower seed skins and excess water.

- Add Soma Salt, Mom's Spice, and a sprinkle of lime juice (optional).

- Blend all together into a medium-thick paste. Put in an air-tight container for storage.

- Serve in individual bowls the same day.

This mixture is as delicious as it is easy to make!

Gymnema Brew Coffee Substitute

Gymnema Brew Coffee Substitute contains Gymnema, Indian Kino, Jamun Seed, Fenugreek, Date Seed, Chicory, and Sweet Cinnamon

- In a covered saucepan, boil six ounces of water mixed with 1 teaspoon of Gymnema powder.

- Do not strain. Do not use sugar. Use almond milk if you like.

This coffee substitute is best consumed before breakfast. It will stimulate your appetite and assist the transformation of glucose.

Precaution: This is a strong formula. Do not use if you have any tendency towards low blood sugar.

Garcinia Tea

Ingredients:

- Garcinia Cambogia, Green Cardamom (Elettaria cardamomum), Cinnamon, Black pepper (Piper nigrum), Nutmeg (Myristica), Fennel (Foeniculum vulgare)

- Use 1 teaspoon of tea and 6 oz of water per person.

- Use a covered saucepan and boil on medium heat for 2-3 minutes.

- Strain and serve.

This SVA Garcinia Tea is tridoshic – balancing for all three doshas. This unique blend of Garcinia with green cardamom pods supports overall metabolism and enhances protein absorption.

Directions for low hunger or no hunger: Drink before breakfast, lunch, and/or dinner. If your hunger is good at meal times, drink this tea after your meals.

Digestive Chutney

Curry leaf
Fresh cilantro
Fresh mint
Soma Salt
Spring Water
Fresh, organic lime, squeezed
Olive Oil (Extra Virgin, cold pressed)

- Clean and chop equal parts curry leaf, cilantro, and mint.

-Place chopped leaves into a small blender and add a little bit of water. Blend into a thin to medium consistency.

-Stir in Soma Salt to tast, add a little bit of olive oil and fresh squeezed lime juice.

Curry leaf is bitter in taste, and very good for the liver and the pancreas. Curry leaves are readily available in Indian grocery stores.

This chutney has an especially wonderful taste and it supports both fat and sugar metabolism, plus it helps to detoxify the blood. You can use it as an accompaniment to any meal, or as a dip.

SVA Moringa Soup

Ingredients: Shade dried bitter moringa leaf powder, arrowroot powder, toasted organic coriander, soma salt, Mom's spice

- Use 1 Tablespoon of soup mix in 8 oz of cool water per serving and mix well.

- Boil 5 minutes in a covered saucepan. Remove from heat,

- Add Soma Salt to taste, a few drops of olive oil, and garnish with chopped cilantro and fresh lime juice.

SVA Moringa Soup mix is delicious eaten as is. For even greater enjoyment add your favorite cooked vegetables to your soup.

Low-Glycemic Salad

Romaine Lettuce (cleaned and chopped)
Cucumber (peeled and chopped)
White Daikon (peeled and chopped)
Mom's Spice
Soma Salt
Olive Oil

- Prepare equal parts of lettuce, cucumber and white daikon. Put in a salad bowl.

- Sprinkle Mom's spice, Soma Salt to taste, and drizzle with olive oil.

- Toss and enjoy!

Tip: Daikon Radish looks like a big white carrot and is available at Indian grocery stores and most specialty grocery stores.

Mom's Spice contains 18 different spices, and they are pre-toasted, so you can sprinkle it straight onto salads, soups or sandwiches. Usually you have to cook with Indian spices, but this blend is pre-toasted so you can use it for flavoring.

Scientific References

Asian Pacific Journal of Tropical Disease, April 2013, pages 93-102

"Antidiabetic effects of *Momordica charantia* (bitter melon) and its medicinal potency"

Baby Joseph: Interdisciplinary Research Center, Department of Biotechnology, Malankara Catholic College, Mariagirl, Kaliakkavilai – 629153, Kanyakumari District, TamilNadu, India

Diabetes Research and Clinical Practice, March 2001, pages 155-161

"Hypotriglyceridemic and hypocholesterolemic effects of anti-diabetic Momordica charantia (karela) fruit extract in streptozotacin-induced diabetic rats.

I. Ahmen, M.S. Lakhani, M. Gillett, A. John, H. Raza: Departments of Anatomy and Biochemistry, Faculty of Medicine and Health Sciences, UAE University, P.O. Box 17666, Al Ain, United Arab Emirates

Journal of Ethnopharmacology, May 1998, Pages 107

"Hypoglucaemic activity of *Syzigium cumini* (jamun) seeds: effect on lipid peroxidation in alloxan diabetic rats"

P. Stanely Mainzen Prince, Venugopal P Menon, L. Pari: Department of Biochemistry, Annamalai University, Annamalai nagar 608 002, Tamil Nadu, India

Molecular Nutrition & Food Research, September 2013, pages 1510-1526

"Multitargeting by turmeric, the golden spice: From kitchen to clinic"

Gupta, S. C., Sung, B., Kim, J. H., Prasad, S., Li, S. and Aggarwal, B. B.

Molecular Nutrition & Food Research, November 2010, pages 1596-1608

"Diosgenin present in fenugreek improves glucose metabolism by promoting adipocyte differentiation and inhibiting inflammation in adipose tissues."

Uemura, T., Hirai, S., Mizoguchi, N., Goto, T., Lee, J.-Y., Taketani, K., Nakano, Y., Shono, J., Hoshino, S., Tsuge, N., Narukami, T., Takahashi, N. and Kawada, T.

Pharmacognosy Review, 2009, pages 359-363

"*Pterocarpus marsupium* Roxb. (Indian Kino) - A comprehensive review"

Manish Devgun, Arun Nanda, SH Ansari

Journal of Ethnopharmacology, October 1990, pages 265-279

"Possible regeneration of the islets of Langerhans in streptozotocin-diabetic rats given gymnema sylvestre leaf extracts"

E.R.B. Shanmugasundaram, K. Leela Gopinath, K. Radha Shanmugasundaram, V.M. Rajendran

Molecular and Cellular Biochemistry, 2007

"Decreased bodyweight without rebound and regulated lipoprotein metabolism by gymnemate in genetic multifactor syndrome animal."

Department of Pathophysiological and Therapeutic Science, Division of Medical Biochemistry, Faculty of Medicine, Tottori University, Yonago, Japan.

International Research Journal of Pharmacy, 2010, pages 100-104

"Phytochemistry and pharmacological activities of *Pterocarpus Marsupium* (Indian Kino) – a Review"

Gairola Seema, Gupta Vikas, Singh Baljinder, Mairhani Mukesh, Bansal PArveen, School of Pharmaceutical Sciences, Shobhit University, Meerut, India, University Centre of Excellence in Research, BFUHS, Fairdkot, India, Department of Biochemistry, PGIMER, Chandigarh, India

About the Authors

Vaidya Ramakant Mishra

Vaidya Mishra is an ayurvedic physician, educator, formulator, researcher, and author, as well as a prolific blogger. 14th in a direct line of ayurvedic physicians to the royalty of India, he was born into the SVA lineage, in Vaidyachak ("village of vaidyas") in the State of Bihar, Northwest India.

Born to an ayurvedic father, Vaidya Kameshwar Mishra, in 1952, his whole life has been imbued and immersed in the research and study of Ayurveda and all its aspects. After graduating from Bihar's SYNA Ayurvedic College in 1974 and earning the title of GAMS (Graduate of Ayurvedic Medicine and Surgery), Vaidya Mishra entered upon an additional intensive seven-year training with his father, the renowned Vaidya Kameshwar Mishra, and was handed over the family and lineage secrets and knowledge. (More information about Vaidya Mishra's lineage can be found in SV Ayurveda, from Sutra to Science, Volume 1, also: www.vaidyamishra.com)

Vaidya Mishra left India to tour Holland and England in 1991. In-between 1991-1996, he toured the United States, Japan, and several European countries. He permanently left India for the United States in 1996. He has since then, lived in the United States, practicing Ayurveda, teaching, and writing.

Vaidya Mishra currently lives in Los Angeles. He is married to Milena Takvorian. You can visit his center, the Prana Center, in Chatsworth, where he practices SV Ayurveda (Shaka Vansiya Ayurveda), offering one-on-one ayurvedic consultations, on-line courses, as well as numerous workshops, talks, conferences. You can view his YouTube channel, SVA Health, for videos. Vaidya Mishra, as a traditional ayurvedic practitioner, also excels at formulations and supplying unique herbal remedies, in supplement or transdermal form, to his clients. For more information, visit his website: www.chandika.com

Lissa Coffey

Lissa Coffey is a lifestyle, relationship and wellness expert who serves up an inspiring blend of ancient wisdom and modern style on her website CoffeyTalk.com and in her e-mail newsletters. She is the host of the popular CoffeyTalk channel on YouTube. Lissa is the author of several books, including the bestselling *What's Your Dosha, Baby? Discover the Vedic Way for Compatibility in Life and Love*. Lissa started her television career at ABC-TV, and went on to run Bamboo Entertainment, Inc., which produces content in nearly every form of media.

A sought-after guest expert, Lissa Coffey appears frequently on television and radio and contributes to many national publications with her insightful and compassionate approach to modern-day issues. Her e-mail newsletters are enjoyed globally by a steadily growing subscriber base. She travels the world giving presentations on her "Ancient Wisdom, Modern Style" philosophy.

Lissa holds degrees and certification in Sociology, Ayurveda, Hypnotherapy and Meditation. Many of her online courses can be found at TransformativeU.com.

Lissa lives in Westlake Village, California with her husband Greg. Between the two of them they have five children. Lissa is a vegan who loves to cook, and many of her recipes are on her website.

Aknowledgements

Deep gratitude to Vaidya Mishra's team at the Prana Center, especially Milena Mishra for her loving enthusiasm and vibrant energy.

Thank you to the Gandhi family for their ongoing support of SV Ayurveda.

Thank you to Lissa's team at CoffeyTalk, especially Greg who is always good at taking care of the details. Much gratitude always to The Vedanta Society of Southern California.

Thank you to our teachers for their wisdom, and to our students for being the channel through which this wisdom will live on.

Resources

SV Ayurveda Products

www.Chandika.com

Vaidya Mishra's Blog

www.vaidyamishra.com/blog

Vaidya Mishra's Site

www.vaidyamishra.com

Lissa Coffey's Websites

www.CoffeyTalk.com

www.WhatsYourDosha.com

Made in the USA
Coppell, TX
27 May 2024

32845359R00069